OBESE NO MORE

FOLLOW MY JOURNEY

Judith Coppe Kersten

Published in Australia by Sid Harta Books & Print Pty Ltd,
ABN: 34632585293
17 Coleman Parade, GLEN WAVERLEY VIC 3150 Australia
Telephone: +61 3 9560 9920, Facsimile: +61 3 9545 1742
E-mail: author@sidharta.com.au

First published in Australia 2020
Second edition published 2021

Copyright © Judith Coppe Kersten 2021

Cover design, typesetting: WorkingType (www.workingtype.com.au)

Coppe Kersten, Judith
Obese No More: Follow My Journey
ISBN: 978-1-925707-23-6
pp108

About the Author

Judith Coppe Kersten is Australian. She was brought up in Cowra NSW. At age 17, she had a calling to become a nurse. Helping people was natural to her. Her general training began in Sydney, marriage followed, then she started a family. She's travelled around Australia and overseas.

Her interest in nutritional food started because she wanted to give her children a healthy life.

Judith is retired and lives in Chittaway Bay, NSW, to be near her family.

Introduction

The discovery of finding the secret to staying at goal weight and stopping yo yo dieting was the inspiration for writing this book The revelation was like a bolt from the blue which is why I want my story to be helpful to those who are struggling with maintaining goal weight

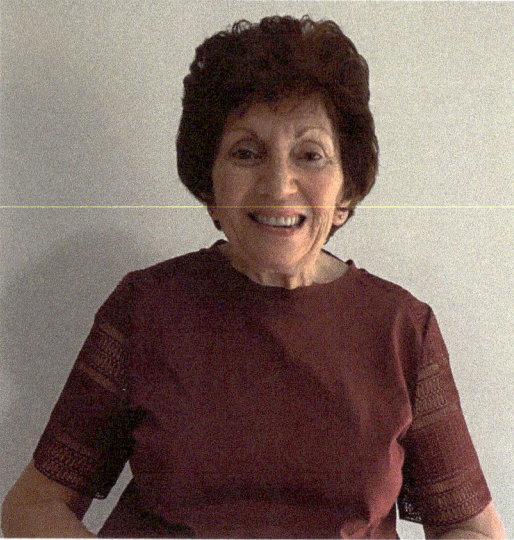

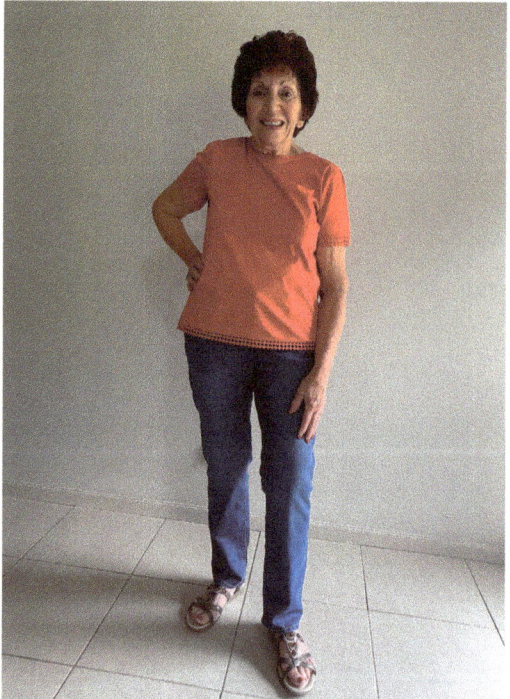

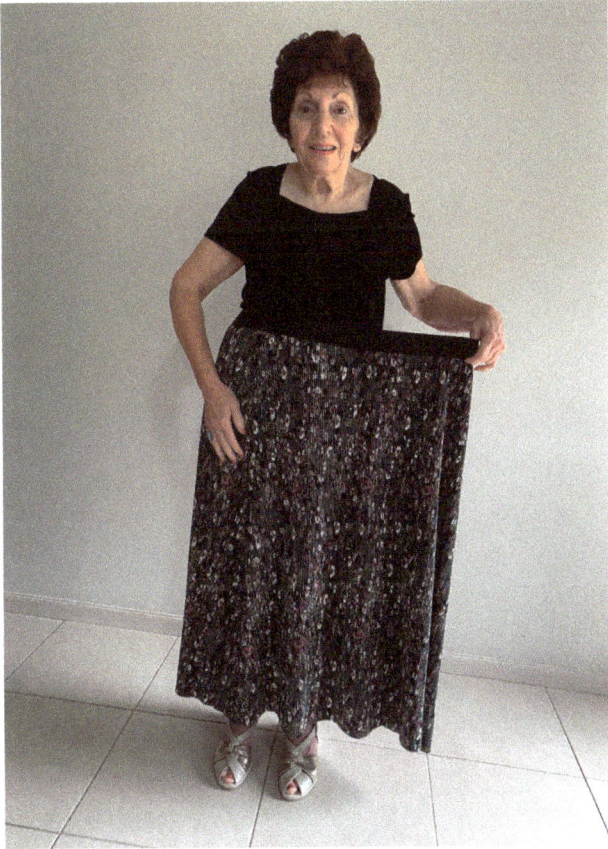

From 94kgs to 70kgs,
and able to wear jeans again!

To my four children
Anthony, Christopher, Paul, Jacqueline.
All of you give purpose to my life
and the inspiration for this book.

Acknowledgements

To my son-in-law Ron Beresford.

Thank you for very patient tutoring in I.T. and the support as I wrote this book.

Preface

Italian Heritage

....

I have Italian heritage from my father Laurence Coppe. I felt a need to go to the country where his parents were born. Before Christmas in 2014, I booked a trip to Italy and left in April 2015. Ahead of me were day trips with groups to see the sights, but also long flights. I became aware of my obesity and thought to myself, 'What have I done?' I cannot do this. This led me to have a big wake-up call. I was obese, unfit, desperate ... help! After I calmed down and became more rational, I needed to put a plan in place. There was a sense of urgency in my life at the time, but I had a goal ... the trip. Christmas was only a few weeks away. The first thing I did decide was that the plan had to start on January 1, 2015. This would give me three and a half months to lose some weight. I had a daydream. You could call it an epiphany. When I thought back to my teenage years, I wished I could be that girl again, slim and energetic. I was a teenager in the 1950s. There was swimming, netball, basketball, tennis and dancing. Oh well, those days were long gone! This was in a small country town called Cowra, NSW. Back then if I didn't do sport, I didn't do anything because there was literally nothing else for me to do. I was exercising a lot without consciously being aware of it or knowing how good it was for me. Also I walked everywhere to get to activities. The natural rhythm for my body was energy in and energy out. I recall that moment of wishful thinking. Now it is 2020 and I have kept at my goal weight of 70kg. The dream finally came true — EUREKA!

CONTENTS

Chapter 1

Health

....

A visit to see my medical doctor was the first step. It was for a check-up on my current health. I was weighed, height measured, blood pressure recorded. She considered my medical history then said that 72 kilos would be a weight to aim for. My immediate thought was that this was impossible! I left the consultation with the word *obese* ringing in my ears. This was a shock. I had never thought of myself as obese. That label was for other people, not me. However, this was my reality: do not lose the plot — lose the weight.

Chapter 2

Obese, Overweight, Fat

....

Whatever the title, the reality was that I was at 94 kilos and I was very uncomfortable. Having difficulty coping with everyday life, like becoming breathless when climbing stairs or going to the letterbox. I had to do housework in short bursts. When I did any gardening, exhaustion set in and I didn't do anything else for the day, except sat. When I dragged myself out to do the shopping, the trolley became a lean-to. As I walked, I was tipping from side to side like an anchored boat. I didn't seem to make any headway. I was very slow getting out of chairs, off toilet seats, out of the car. I could have done with a hoist. Having a bath was ruled out after the day I got trapped ... the oil in the water didn't help. The towel wound around the tap to make a pulley and I was able to pull myself up eventually and literally rolled over the side of the bath. My breast size increased, and I considered a surgical reduction. I only wore bras when I left the house because by the afternoon my bra felt like a tight brace and couldn't be tolerated. Friction on the inner thighs caused me redness and discomfort. Talcum powder gave relief. My legs felt like logs with feet attached and the pouffe became my best friend. Obesity is no laughing matter.

Chapter 3

Observations

....

When people do not see each other for a long time, they notice changes. My mother came to stay with us for a month in the 1970s. She was walking behind me one day when she remarked that I was getting a bit "hippy". She didn't mean I was alternative as in the 1970's hippy movement. She had seen I had a broad beam, a big backside, and a bottom that went boom, boom as I walked. This made me aware that I had put on weight and then began the journey of yoyo dieting over the years. In short, I became a weight-watch tragic. You name it, I tried it over the years hoping for a magic fix.

- Weight watch groups
- Tablets to suppress appetite

- Food bars to replace meals
- Powder to make shakes and replace meals
- Capsules to take before meals to absorb fat
- Diet meals prepared for a week by companies and delivered to my home.

The only thing I lost was a truckload of money. Starting something new always became my New Year resolution. Whatever I did, it always had a short timeframe because I was missing my own food choices and craving to eat the food that my brain was hard-wired to eat. As a child, I can recall my experiences of food and drinks my mother cooked and served for the family. The aromas wafting through our house are forever cemented in my memory. Roast beef and vegetables with hot puddings and hot drinks are still my favourite during the winter. In summer, we had salads, cold meats, cold drinks and desserts.

On a cold day, when I felt cold, my body told me to put more clothes on. It was also telling me that I needed more energy to keep warm and to eat hot food and drinks. On a hot day when I felt hot, my body told me to only wear light clothing. It was also telling me

I needed less energy, so to help keep cool, I needed to have cool food and cold drinks.

Mother was right. She did not have to be told this was a natural way to eat and drink. She had a saying: 'Money is better spent on wholesome food,' and 'An apple a day keeps the doctor away'.

Eventually there came a time when I discontinued the diet meals delivery. It wasn't economical. I still had to shop and cook for 5 other family members and they didn't really understand why I was eating different food to them. My weight would then increase, but I did not know how to manage it myself, i.e. calculate the daily calorie count.

Chapter 4

Delay

....

Delaying to lose weight and putting doing it on hold, always resulted in me gaining even more weight. Eating and drinking with reckless abandon and thinking that weight will come off when it's the right time for me to start shedding it, was a mindset I had to change. The realisation came when I realised that my weight, 70 kilos, had to be interwoven with everyday life. My daily calorie count had to become 1200 calories.

Chapter 5

Procrastination — The thief of time

The queen of procrastination lives here. Delaying and postponing what I have to do and sitting down and just thinking became a habit of mine. The less I did, the more I didn't want to do. Boredom set in. The cravings for something sweet became a habit. Circulation became slow, so when I did get up from a chair, there was a delay to get walking. By not focusing on activities, it was lunchtime before anything got done. I had to tackle this problem. I tried a different approach and listed tasks on a notepad at breakfast time. This gave me purpose and made me keep moving, only stopping for meals. Gardening, walking, swimming, shopping, housework; houses are unforgiving there's always things to do. At the end of the day I ticked off the tasks. It's surprising how good it is to see how much is achieved. If there's still tasks left, they carry over to the next day. The more I did, the more I wanted to do. A big success towards losing kilos and getting to goal weight. The list became longer — painting the house was never on the list!

Chapter 6

Energy in, Energy out

As I am driving my car I have a light-globe moment. I stop at the service station to fill up my car. The analogy is that my car needs petrol. If the fuel tank is filled beyond capacity, there is overflow onto my feet. Not a pleasant experience. The same can be said for my body. If I eat more food than my body actually needs, it overflows and becomes fat. Driving the car burns the fuel, it's similar to exercise — it burns the fuel i.e. the food that I eat. Now every time I go to the service station to get petrol, I don't overfill the tank. The same with the food I put into my body: do not overfill, do not overeat. My car parked in the garage is not burning fuel. When I'm sitting in a chair, I am not burning fat. I do not give my body any more food than it needs.

Chapter 7

Exercise

....

There is no typical day for me. Exercise is interwoven with activities that crop up. They could be shopping, swimming, school pick-ups, going to walking at the park, etc.

There are a lot of opportunities to move about. If the phone rings I do not sit but walk around as I talk. The movement all adds up.

For school pick-ups, I park the car a street or two away from the school.

Shopping at the Mall is basically window shopping, as I walk around for 30 to 45 minutes.

Walking in a sheltered place is good for wet days and also when it's too hot outside.

I pack a bag for swimming or walking and always take a bottle of water.

Having the bag ready saves me time so that I don't have to look for items. This gets me out of the house quickly.

Chapter 8

Sleep Apnoea

....

Sleep Apnoea is a medical condition I didn't know I was suffering from for years. It was partially the reason I was eating the wrong food, so that I could stay more alert during the day. Sweet sugary foods and high carbohydrate foods are all very nice to eat, but unfortunately they were also contributing to me becoming overweight. Snoring and irregular breathing was preventing me from going into a deep sleep. It was a constant interruption to my sleep pattern at night. So, I was waking up in the morning feeling sluggish physically and with a brain fog similar to jetlag. This lasted for about two-thirds of the day and falling asleep after lunch was a regular occurrence. Appointments were always made in the afternoon and I told people that 'I'm not a morning person.' I was not functioning properly because I had Sleep Apnoea.

Chapter 9

Fat as protection

....

A partner who was jealous and possessive and also passive-aggressive caused me to have emotional problems. I felt isolated from family and friends because he questioned everything I said or did. Not resisting that attitude gave me a more peaceful day, however I felt underlying anger. Love for food became a comfort and my weight increased. By wearing no makeup and having just plain clothes, I felt invisible and safe. I didn't attract attention. I wasn't getting interrogated. When I was on my own at 47, I felt free to be myself. I still had emotional problems, so overeating and yoyo dieting were ongoing. I still had a fear of looking too good, getting the wrong attention and being self-conscious. I have now finally overcome this, but it has taken many years. One Christmas when I had reached goal-weight, my teenage granddaughter said to me: 'NANNY YOU LOOK AMAZING'. I felt as if I had just graduated. My mantra now is, 'I'm never too old to look and feel good.'

I am woman, I am strong!

Chapter 10

Hindsight

....

I looked back to when I was married and had 4 children under 7. In hindsight, I wish I had not neglected my appearance. I can remember there were days I didn't look in the mirror because I was so busy. I became tired and dull and lost all feeling about myself. I became invisible. I had a sudden interest in my appearance and losing weight. I thought to myself, 'If I don't do it for me, who am I doing it for?'

I realised that even while in a relationship, it was important to make time for myself. It does take an effort. Looking back, it seemed impossible because the daylight hours went so fast. Therefore, meeting him at the front door with the castanets and the rose between my teeth was never going to happen.

Chapter 11

Hygiene

....

Over the years I noticed birds and animals preen themselves in the early part of the day. This has given me the idea that early is the best time to attend to myself and to feel better able to face the day. A regime was necessary, simple and basic was the way to go. If I jump into the day and lunch rolls around and I haven't done this, I felt daggy and vulnerable. Getting clothes out the night before saved me time. No hesitation to get dressed. My regime is: shower, use deodorant, clean teeth, moisturise face, tidy hair, apply lipstick, check fingernails. No matter how the day goes, I am ready for it. I would go to the letterbox and answer the doorbell with confidence. I had a reminder to never leave my house in a dressing gown and nightie after this happened one morning: I did a drop-off to the railway station and halfway back to the house I ran out of petrol. My neighbour had also dropped someone off and I saw him approaching, so I jumped in his car hoping the neighbours were too busy to look out the window when I got out of the car red-faced.

Chapter 12

Clothes Sizes

....

As my weight reduced, my clothes size changed over the year that it took me to reach my goal weight. A few trips to the charity shop to drop off the bigger sizes felt good. No emotional attachment. Out they went. I didn't keep them in case I gained weight again and couldn't find anything in my wardrobe that would fit me. Over the years I had a collection of clothes that ranged in sizes:

24, 22, 20, 18, 16, 14, 12 and nothing was fashionable. When I did shop for my weight I would buy clothes at sales that were not expensive; I just needed a fresh look.

I found the best way is to divide my wardrobe into

clothes for activities. So I have clothes for at home, smart-casual for being out and about, dress-up clothes for semi and formal occasions. I now feel I don't have to wait for special occasions to feel good about myself and to feel well-dressed most of the time. People will recognise my way of describing this as getting out the 'glad rags'. We don't always need to be going out to enjoy wearing nice clothes. Obviously, I don't get out the ball gown to do the gardening.

Chapter 13

Clothes — appearance

Don't you just love the change room mirrors in the stores? The funny mirrors at Luna Park are more flattering. I started to avoid going into them. So the solution for me was to buy garments and try them on at home. Whoever designed the tent dresses and track suits must of had me in mind. I loved them. In the 1980s and 1990s, these were the clothes everyone was wearing. But the line was drawn for me at size 24. Checking out the maternity section during sales I realised it was not a good idea, as my self-esteem was already at rock bottom. When I had lost some weight, I found I could fit into size 18. This was exciting because the shops were starting to display fashionable clothes in the bigger sizes. This was the start for me to look better and feel better. I booked a stylist at the department store and she selected a classic mix-and-match set of clothes as a foundation for my wardrobe that I could add more pieces to. I did this for the winter and summer clothes. The family couldn't believe how good I looked. This gave me a lot of confidence. As the weight came off, my size went down. The money I saved from not overeating, I bought new clothes with. I didn't wait. Size 18 became size 16 and then size 14 and I even have some clothes in my wardrobe sized 12. January 2015, I was 94 kilos, by October 2015, I was 70 kilos and in 2020, I managed to stay at 70 kilos. These days, shopping for clothes has become enjoyable.

Chapter 14

Deprivation

....

Feeling deprived is the enemy of successful weight loss and for staying at goal weight. It can also eventually lead me to start binging. The craving can be for sweet or savoury food. It can happen if I am really hungry and if I have not had time to prepare the meals and snacks for the day. This can be triggered by advertisements or the aromas wafting from food outlets and restaurants. When the food is on display, the pull is powerful.

If it is summer, my cravings are for something sweet. When I have the sweet craving it can be for example, ice cream and salted caramel sauce with a dollop of double cream or apple pie, custard and cream, the list goes on.

My winter cravings are savoury, like meat pies, sausage rolls with tomato sauce. I can actually feel my body reacting to overeating and I can feel borderline sick. This puts me off eating food for the rest of the day. This is instead of a meal. I call it ...THE SWITCHEROO.

Giving in to cravings is definitely the way to go. It satisfies me for a while making sure that I do not have cravings for a long time. Fear of food is a burden I do not need. I keep a good variety of sweet and savoury food in the fridge, freezer and pantry. It is available for next time.

There was a man who had a lolly shop. He said to his new employee: Eat as many lollies as you feel like. She did this for some days to the point where she did not eat another lolly. He was wise to say that to her. This story rings bells.

Chapter 15

Enjoyment

....

Life should be enjoyed. Eating and drinking plays a very important part. After all, we need it to sustain life.

The secret is not to make it my enemy. I know now that I can have all food that I want, but just not all at once.

It does not make any sense to me when I hear that any one food or drink is the magic fix to losing weight.

Example: Powder sachets/shakes
Example: Grapefruit

I do not force myself to have anything that is not to my taste just because it may make me lose weight.

It is the variety of food I select for the day, keeping in mind not to go over 1200 calories.

Keeping the pantry fridge and freezer well-stocked with a good variety of food and drinks is a good idea to choose from each day.

Keeping a notepad on the kitchen bench is essential. I jot down items that I am close to finishing and this makes shopping a lot easier.

Chapter 16

Busy Me

....

The checks and balances are all too consuming and it seems difficult to keep weight under control and remain healthy. Then I have this voice in my head: wait a minute, I would spend more time and money on ill health and visits to doctors if I remained unhealthy. A good wake-up call for my reasoning to not put the cart before the horse. After all, the horse has to be healthy to pull the cart. There can be days ahead that need planning, so that a busy day does not turn into a grab fest: see it, eat it. Prepare the meals the night before. Cook extra the night before to reheat for dinner, or have in the freezer a low calorie meal as a good quick-fix if you haven't prepared ahead. Also, the tote bag comes out for packing morning tea, lunch and afternoon tea if I'm away from home.

Tote bag list e.g. for morning tea, lunch and afternoon tea:

- 2 low-calorie sweet biscuits
- A sandwich
- 1 bottle of water
- 1 piece of fruit
- 1 takeout skinny coffee

This enables me to mix and match the food and drink as the day rolls on. Also, 1 paper serviette, 1 plastic fork and spoon if I buy a yoghurt or pasta from the shop. If I haven't packed a tote bag, I usually buy a bun with salad, meat or fish. The calorie count for this item is displayed on the packaging or on the board if bought at the counter. So, the calorie count consumed for morning tea, lunch and afternoon tea is added to the breakfast calories and then deducted from the 1200 daily calories, so that the final balance are the calories allowed for my dinner. I would love to see all food outlets and restaurants display on their menus a total amount of calories when selecting food to buy. It would make it easier to fit it into my 1200 calorie count for the day. The solution is to take my calorie count book and calculator.

Chapter 17

Water

....

Hydration is important for circulation. I know my body is 70% or more of water, so a good balance of fluid in my body must be maintained and replaced. Each morning a 2-litre jug is filled with filtered water for the day to stay on the kitchen bench as a reminder to drink. I like water at room temperature drunk from a glass with a straw. It means I can consume it faster. Also, from the jug, I fill the kettle for tea and coffee and bottles to take when I leave the house. Plus, I have a bottle of water in the bathroom with a glass and a straw. A glass of water before meals is a good thing to do to reduce appetite, and by the end of the day, the jug on the bench is usually empty.

Chapter 18

Sugar fat salt

....

For quite a few years now, I stopped adding sugar to tea and coffee and it took me some time to get used to the taste. I did it by gradually adding less each time, so eventually I did not add it at all.

Having any food where I would add sugar to cereal, e.g. Weetbix or porridge, a gradual reduction gave me the same results. This is also the same with fat. When I am at the shops I look for fat-reduced food, e.g. dairy foods: 99% skim milk, 99% low fat yoghurt and low fat cheese, etc. Reducing added salt can also be done. I no longer add salt to my food. I also select no added salt in packaged or tin food. Awareness of sugar, fat and salt content in most food at the shops and making sure that everything is selected with a critical eye is the key. The changeover was time consuming, but it is now automatic. I now know which products I need to buy. There are no longer the feelings of a guilt trip, apprehension or confusion. Dare I say it? Shopping has become a pleasure.

Keeping to the 1200 calorie count of food for the day, results in a natural reduction. Sugar, salt and fat become a lot lower.

Chapter 19

Notebook

....

A notebook is kept in the kitchen for recording the food and drink I have in the fridge, freezer and pantry. This is my quick go-to for weights and calories of food I am preparing. Each food group is listed on a different page with a column of weight and a column for calories.

The groups are:

Dairy plus eggs, meat, fish, fruit, vegetables plus salad, cereal plus bread, snacks, drinks, spreads plus sauces, confectionery.

Chapter 20

Calculating calories

....

Tools

- 1 digital kitchen scale
- 1 calculator
- Book — calorie, fat and carbohydrate counter

Every day there are numbers to crunch. Incidentally it is good for the brain. Simple arithmetic like multiplication, addition, subtraction and division is what I apply. The food I am preparing for breakfast, morning tea, lunch, afternoon tea, appetizer and dinner is weighed, and calories are counted. If it is in kilojoules, I divide that number by 4.2 which equals calories.

E.g. 100kj divided by 4.2 = 24 Calories

Calculations ending in a decimal point are rounded up to the next calorie.

Weighing food is essential to calculate calories.

Fruit

Orange — e.g. remove skin 50g = 20 calories
Vegetables — e.g. zucchini 63g = 8 calories

Wrap remainder in cling wrap and place in fridge.

Packaged food:

Check panel.

Marie biscuits e.g. 2 biscuits 12g = 54 calories

Tinned food 110g tin of sardines in spring water e.g. 75g = 133 calories

Put remainder in dish, cover and place in the fridge

Smaller portions allow a bigger variety of food for the day

All food and drinks have a calorie value. Weigh vegetables plus meat to get a calorie count for a meal. Be mindful of dressings, sauces and gravy which often have a high calorie count.

Tip: Steam vegetables

Chapter 21

Mix and Match

....

Creative thinking is what is needed to mix and match food. I leave complicated cooking to the professionals. At home, simple is best and quicker to prepare meals. Separating ingredients to put a meal together, allows me to add up calories. The variety of food in the fridge, freezer and pantry is based on the following food groups:

- Dairy
- Eggs
- Meats
- Fish
- Fruit
- Vegetables
- Cereals and bread

I am only limited by my own imagination to create meals.

To demonstrate how I calculate 1200 Calories for my daily way of eating, here are seven examples of meals and snacks that add up to 1200 calories.

EXAMPLE 1

Breakfast

Food selected

- Bread
- 1 box Weetbix
- Long-life skim milk
- Packet of low-fat sliced cheese
- Jar Vegemite
- Jar smooth peanut butter
- Jar marmalade jam
- Tea

Create Meal

Breakfast:

Grams		Calories
59	2 slices of bread	143
15	1 Weetbix	54
250 ml of skim milk daily allowance		88
1 slice of cheese		41
1/2 tsp of Vegemite		5

1/2 teaspoon of peanut butter	15
1 teaspoon marmalade jam	15
Tea	Nil
Total =	361 calories

Morning Tea:

Food selected

1 packet of Marie biscuits
1 punnet strawberries

Food	Calories
2 Marie biscuits	54
75g strawberries	20
Coffee	0
Total:	74 calories

Lunch

Food selected:

- 1 tin sardines in spring water
- 1 lettuce
- 1 tomato
- 1 cucumber
- 1 can beetroot
- 1 onion
- 1 red capsicum
- Low-fat French dressing
- Jar tartare sauce
- Kiwi fruit

Create Meal

Grams		Calories
75	Sardines	133
30	Lettuce	5
75	Tomato	15
50	Cucumber	5
30	Beetroot	15
30	Onion	10
1 tbsp	French dressing	17

5	Tartare sauce	30
100	Kiwi fruit	40
		Total: 270 Calories

Afternoon Tea

Food selected for Afternoon Tea

1 packet shortbread cream biscuits

1 packet caramel cream lollies

Food	Calories
1 shortbread cream biscuit	85
1 caramel cream lolly	25
Tea/coffee	nil
Total:	110 Calories

Appetizer

Food	Calories
150mls Dry white wine	94
40g Tzatziki dip	42
3 fine wafer crackers	20
Total:	156 calories

Dinner

Food selected:

1 packet veal leg steak

1 bottle tomato sauce

Carrots

Zucchini

Snow peas

Green beans

Broccoli

Butter

Create Meal:

Grams		Calories
100	veal leg steak	110
50	carrot	15
63	zucchini	8
33	snow peas	10
30	green beans	10
45	broccoli	15
1 tsp	butter	35
1 tbsp	tomato sauce	25
Total:		228 calories

TOTAL FOR THE DAY

	Calories
Breakfast	361 +
Morning Tea	74 +
Lunch	270 +
Afternoon Tea	110 +
Appetizer	156 +
Dinner	228 +
Total =	1200 Calories approximately

Example 2

Breakfast

Food selected

Bread

Porridge (rolled oats)

Long-life skim milk

Jar Vegemite

Jar honey

Tea

Create meal:

Breakfast

Grams		Calories
59	2 slices of bread	143
25	Rolled oats	100
250 ml of skim milk daily allowance		88
1 tsp honey		20
½ tsp Vegemite		5
Tea		Nil
Total:		356 calories

Food selected for Morning Tea:

1 packet of Milk arrowroot biscuits
1 mandarin

Morning Tea:

	Calories
1 Milk Arrowroot biscuit	35
80g mandarin	30
Coffee	Nil
Total:	65 calories

Lunch

Food selected:

1 Pkt bread rolls

1 Pkt fat-free turkey slices

1 lettuce

1 tomato

1 cucumber

1 can beetroot

1 onion

Fat-free mayonnaise

Create Meal:

Grams		Calories
75	Bread roll	190
40g	Turkey slices	42
20	Lettuce	2
45	Tomato	8
25	Cucumber	3
18	Beetroot	10
10	Onion	3
1 dsp	Mayonnaise	12
Total:		270 Calories

Afternoon Tea

Food selected:

1 packet Iced Vovo biscuits
1 packet Fantales lollies

	Calories
1 Iced Vovo biscuit	55
1 Fantales lolly	30
Tea/coffee	nil
Total:	85 Calories

Appetizer

	Calories
150mls Dry white wine	94
40g Tzatziki Dip	42
4 fine wafer crackers	25
Total:	161 calories

Dinner

Food selected:

Atlantic salmon

Lettuce

Avocado

Tomato

Cucumber

Fat-free French dressing

Lemon juice

Tartare sauce

Create meal:

Grams		Calories
75	Atlantic salmon	140
20	Lettuce	2
75	Tomato	15
50	Cucumber	5
20	Avocado	43
1 tbsp fat-free French dressing		17
1 tsp Tartare sauce		30
30mls Lemon juice		10
Total		262 calories

TOTAL FOR THE DAY

	Calories
Breakfast	356 +
Morning Tea	65 +
Lunch	270 +
Afternoon Tea	85 +
Appetizer	161 +
Dinner	262 +
Total	1200 Calories approximately

Example 3

Breakfast

Food selected

Bread

Egg

Long-life skim milk

Jar peanut butter

Jar apricot jam

Tea

Create meal:

Grams		Calories
59	2 slices of bread	143
48	Egg	70
250 ml of skim milk daily allowance		88
1 tsp peanut butter		30
1 tsp apricot jam		15
Tea		Nil
Total:		346 calories

Food selected for Morning Tea:

1 packet of Milk Coffee biscuits
White grapes
Coffee

	Calories
1 Milk Coffee biscuit	35
40g White grapes	25
Coffee	Nil
Total:	80 calories

Lunch

Food selected:

1 can fat-free chunky chicken soup
Bread
1 pkt fat-free sliced cheese
1 Kiwi fruit

Create Meal:

Grams		Calories
250	Soup	131
30	1 slice bread	72
1 slice cheese		41
100	Kiwi fruit	40
Total:		284 calories

Afternoon Tea

Food selected:

1 packet shortbread biscuits

1 packet butterscotch lollies

Coffee/tea

	Calories
1 Shortbread biscuit	60
1 Butterscotch lolly	25
Tea/coffee	nil
Total:	85 Calories

Appetizer

	Calories
150 mls Red wine	100
10g French onion dip	23
3 fine wafer crackers	20
Total:	143 calories

Dinner

Food selected:

Lean beef steak

White potato

Carrot

Snow peas

Broccoli

Green Beans

Butter

1 Pkt brown onion gravy

Create meal:

Grams		Calories
100	Lean steak	120
50	Potato	35
50	Carrot	15
33	Snow peas	10
45	Broccoli	15
30	Green Beans	10
1 tsp Butter		35
55	Gravy	20
Total:		260 calories

TOTAL FOR THE DAY

	Calories
Breakfast	346 +
Morning Tea	80 +
Lunch	284 +
Afternoon Tea	85 +
Appetizer	143 +
Dinner	260 +
Total:	1200 calories approximately

Example 4

Breakfast

Food selected

Bread
Box crunchy nut clusters
Long-life skim milk
Jar Vegemite
Pkt low-fat sliced cheese
Jar marmalade jam
Tea

Create meal:

Grams		Calories
59	2 slices of bread	143
20	Crunchy nut clusters	83
250 ml of skim milk daily allowance		88
1 slice cheese		41
½ tsp Vegemite		5
1 tsp marmalade jam		15
Tea		Nil
Total:		375 calories

Food selected Morning Tea:

1 packet of Marie biscuits
1 Apricot
Coffee/tea

	Calories
2 Marie biscuits	54
1 60g apricot	20
Coffee/tea	Nil
Total:	74 calories

Lunch

Food selected:

1 fat-free yoghurt
Jar of honey
1 Banana
Walnuts

Create Meal:

Grams		Calories
50	Fat-free yoghurt	80
70g	Banana	100
1 tsp honey		17
8	Walnuts	50
Total:		247 Calories

Afternoon Tea

Food selected:

1 packet Butternut snap biscuits
1 packet butterscotch lollies
Coffee/tea

	Calories
1 Butternut snap biscuit	55
1 Butterscotch lolly	25
Tea/coffee	nil
Total:	80 Calories

Appetizer

	Calories
120mls Dry white wine	75
30g Tzatziki dip	28
3 fine wafer crackers	20
Total:	123 calories

Dinner

Food selected:

Lean chicken breast (skinless)

White potato

Pumpkin

Snap peas

Green Beans

Bottle mild chilli sauce

Create meal:

Grams		Calories
100	Lean chicken breast	150
100	white potato	70
100 pumpkin		45
30 snap peas		10
30	green beans	10
1 tbsp mild chilli sauce		10
Total:		295 calories

TOTAL FOR THE DAY

	Calories
Breakfast	375 +
Morning Tea	74 +
Lunch	247 +
Afternoon Tea	80 +
Appetizer	123 +
Dinner	295 +
Total:	1200 calories approximately

Example 5

Breakfast

Food selected

Bread

Egg

Long-life skim milk

Jar Vegemite

1 pkt low-fat cheese

1 jar honey

Tea

Create meal:

Grams		Calories
59	2 slices of bread	143
45	1 egg	70
250 ml of skim milk daily allowance		88
1 slice cheese		41
½ tsp Vegemite		5
1 tsp honey		20
Tea	Nil	
Total:		367 calories

Morning Tea

Food selected Morning Tea:

1 packet of shredded wheatmeal biscuits

1 punnet strawberries

	Calories
2 shredded wheatmeal Biscuits	60
75g strawberries	20
Coffee /tea	Nil
Total:	80 calories

Lunch

Food selected:

1 can red salmon

1 lettuce

Tomato

Cucumber

Onion

Red capsicum

1 can beetroot

Lemon juice

Low-fat French dressing

1 pear

Create Meal:

Grams		Calories
40	Red salmon	65
30g	Lettuce	5
75	Tomato	15
30	Onion	10
30	Red capsicum	7
50	Cucumber	5
30	Beetroot	15
1 tsp	Lemon juice	15
1 tsp	French dressing	6
115	Pear	65

Total: 208 Calories

Afternoon Tea

<u>Food selected:</u>

1 packet Nice biscuits

1 packet Bon Bon lollies

Coffee/tea

	Calories
1 Nice biscuit	55
1 Bon Bon lolly	20
Tea/coffee	nil
Total:	75 Calories

Appetizer

	Calories
150mls Dry white wine	94
10g French onion dip	23
3 fine wafer crackers	20
Total	137 calories

Dinner

Food selected:

Lamb loin chop

Onion

White potato

Broccoli

Carrot

Snow peas

1 Pkt Brown onion gravy

Create meal:

Grams		Calories
100	Lamb loin chop	200
20	Onion	6
100	White potato	70
45	Broccoli	15
25	Carrot	8
33	Snow Peas	10
55	Brown onion gravy	20
Total:		329 calories

TOTAL FOR THE DAY

	Calories
Breakfast	367 +
Morning Tea	80 +
Lunch	208 +
Afternoon Tea	75 +
Appetizer	137 +
Dinner	329 +
Total	1200 Calories approximately

Example 6

Breakfast

Food selected

Bread

1 box of Weetbix

Long-life skim milk

Jar peanut butter

Low-fat sliced cheese

Jar apricot jam

Tea

Create meal:

Grams		Calories
59	2 slices of bread	143
15	1 Weetbix	54
250 ml of skim milk daily allowance		88
1 slice cheese		41
1 tsp peanut butter		30
1 tsp apricot jam		15
Tea		Nil
Total:		371 calories

Morning Tea

Food selected Morning Tea:

1 packet of wafer biscuits

1 peach

Coffee/tea

Morning Tea:

	Calories
4 wafer Biscuits	40
60g peach	25
Coffee/tea	Nil
Total:	65 calories

Lunch

Food selected:

Bread

Butter

1 can baked beans

1 pkt low-fat cheese

1 orange

Create Meal:

Grams		Calories
59	2 slices bread	143
53	Baked beans	24
1 slice cheese		41
1 tsp butter		35
50	Orange	20
Total:		263 Calories

Afternoon Tea

Food selected:

1 packet Monte biscuits
1 packet caramel cream lollies
Tea/coffee

Afternoon Tea

	Calories
1 Monte biscuit	60
1 Caramel cream lolly	25
Tea/coffee	nil
Total	85 calories

Appetizer

	Calories
375mls Diet dry gingerale	5
1 slice lite tasty cheese	70
4 fine wafer crackers	25
Total:	100 calories

Dinner

Food selected:

Lean pork chop

Sweet red potato

Cauliflower

Snap peas

Broccoli

Zucchini

Apple sauce

Butter

Create meal:

Grams		Calories
150	Lean pork chop	173
50	Sweet potato	33
50	Cauliflower	10
50	Snap peas	10
45	Broccoli	15
34	Zucchini	4
1 tsp butter		35
1 tbsp apple sauce		30
Total		310 calories

TOTAL FOR THE DAY

	Calories
Breakfast	371 +
Morning Tea	65 +
Lunch	263 +
Afternoon Tea	85 +
Appetizer	100 +
Dinner	310 +
Total	1200 Calories approximately

Example 7:

Breakfast

Food selected

Bread

Egg

Long-life skim milk

Low-fat eye-rasher bacon

Jar Vegemite

Jar marmalade jam

Tea

Create meal:

Breakfast:

Grams	Calories
59	2 slices of bread	143
48	Egg	70
250 ml of skim milk daily allowance	88
40 Bacon	55
1/2 tsp Vegemite	5
1 tsp marmalade jam	15
Tea	Nil
Total	376 calories

Morning Tea

Food selected Morning Tea:

1 packet of chocolate finger biscuits
1 orange
Coffee/tea

	Calories
2 Chocolate finger biscuits	64
50g orange	20
Coffee/tea	Nil
Total:	84 calories

Lunch

Food selected:

1 thin crust supreme pizza
1 pkt coleslaw mix
Fat-free coleslaw dressing
1 can pineapple thins

Create Meal:

Lunch

Grams		Calories
70	Sliced pizza	160
85	Coleslaw mix	15
1 tbsp fat-free coleslaw dressing		30
1 slice pineapple thins		25
Total:		230 Calories

Afternoon Tea

Food selected:

1 packet custard cream biscuits

1 packet jelly beans lollies

Coffee/tea

	Calories
1 Custard Cream biscuit	75
2 Jelly bean lollies	10
Tea/coffee	nil
Total:	85 Calories

Appetizer

	Calories
250mls glass diet tonic water	Nil
20g Hummus dip	53
3 fine wafer crackers	20
Total:	73 calories

Dinner

Food selected:

Barramundi fish fillet

White potato

Lettuce

Tomato

Onion

Can corn kernels

Can pineapple thins

Lemon juice

Create meal:

Grams		Calories
150	Barramundi fish fillet	135
150	White potato	105
20	Lettuce	2
10	Onion	3
38	Corn kernels	28
1 slice	pineapple thins	25
1 tsp	lemon juice	15
Total:		342 calories

TOTAL FOR THE DAY

	Calories
Breakfast	376 +
Morning Tea	84 +
Lunch	230 +
Afternoon Tea	85 +
Appetizer	73 +
Dinner	342 +
Total	1200 Calories approximately

Chapter 22

Managing Alcohol

....

Liking a glass of wine three or four evenings a week is something I enjoy, but it unfortunately will increase my weight. It was a big no. It had to stop for at least three months. I was comforting myself with the thought of a reward of my very first glass of wine when I was up and away heading overseas. Anyway, that reward was earlier. A week before the trip, I decided that I deserved my reward because the weight loss was going so well. As a solution to my regular happy hour, while I sustained from alcohol, the wine glass still came out at the end of the day. Instead of wine, I replaced it with diet tonic water or diet ginger ale — the drinks I have when not having alcohol, and a calorie counted snack which was dry biscuits with low-fat cheese.

Chapter 23

Humour: A tribute to my mother Alice Coppe:

....

While recalling the early years as a child with four siblings, during the 1940s and 1950s, my mother always looked on the bright side of life. There always seemed to be something to have a laugh about. If there was anything perceived as gloomy, she would say, 'birds and flowers' as a way of dismissing an atmosphere of unhappiness. My sense of seeing the funny side of life, if I look back, could be attributed to her. It is a legacy I value. Laughter is the best medicine of all ... have fun.

Chapter 24

The Swinging Kilo

....

With my weekends busy with social activities, the Monday weigh-in will usually show an increase in weight. I do not go into panic mode. I have my secret weapon, the swinging kilo. When the 70 kilos goal weight was achieved, I knew I needed some social space, so 71 kilos was in sight. This meant I now had a one kilo range — 70-71 kilos for social occasions. There can be all sorts of celebrations; Christmas, New Year, Easter, birthdays, holidays, dinners and the occasional fast food. You name it, there always seems to be something on. The list is endless. I can have a great weekend, then make time for exercise and counting calories.

Chapter 25

Holiday

....

I go on holidays twice during the year. While I am away from my home, I leave with the intention of having a good time. I love to free range. Eating out is a part of it and do not forget the drinks. Exercise is incidental, as is walking to see parts of the area I happen to be in. Having said that, I still consider portions of food to eat and how often I eat them. The drinks are always plenty of water. This is the best way to quench thirst and sometimes a glass of wine at dinner.

After I lost the kilos and reached my goal weight, my stomach had shrunk and as it happened, I had a lesser capacity for consuming large amounts of food. The week I arrived home, I brought out the scales to weigh myself and noticed that my weight would usually have increased from 1 kilo to 2 kilos. This is what I expected. This is where my swinging kilo kicked in and saved me from anxiety and stress. It was then that I went back on the wagon of counting calories and weighing food and exercising. Move, move, move! Before I know it, the weight gradually comes off.

Chapter 26

Track weight

....

Weighing myself every morning after going to the toilet and before breakfast was really very clear for me. After a big social weekend of not counting calories and of consuming a lot of yummy food, the scales on Monday morning showed that I had gained 1 kilo. The reality wasn't easy to accept. I love vegetables, so it was my go-to solution to have a variety of steamed vegetables and fish for the next 2 days. On Wednesday, my weigh-in showed that I was a kilo less. This showed me how important the daily weigh in is. It has become so important, because while reading my body, I can immediately take action to stop the weight creeping up. Getting to the desired weight is easy, staying there is the hard part.

Chapter 27

The 4 Ws

....

Rising out of bed for the day I have adopted the following daily routine:

- Wee/empty my bladder
- Weigh/bare weight (Remove clothes)
- Write my weight in the book I keep in the bathroom
- Watch/listen to my body

If my weight has gone up, I don't make it a guilt trip. This is my way of recognising what my body is telling me. I ask myself: Did I have a heavy meal the night before? Or did I have too much fluid and no exercise the day before? If I haven't had a bowel movement for one or two days it can also show an increase in weight. The daily routine of the 4 Ws over the last 5 years gives me a simple insight into how my body is functioning each day. This helps me to recognise any corrections that need to be done for the day, e.g. exercise and increase fibre for bowel movements. I am aware of how easy it is for weight to creep in as it has happened to me on numerous occasions. I was able to get to a weight I was happy with, and then before I knew it, the scales showed me an increase in weight. This is why I know I have to be vigilant now.

Chapter 28

Chef, Finances, Illusion

I am not in the position to have a chef in the kitchen. Dinner — a store-bought frozen main meal with a side salad is my go-to when the day has ended, and no food is prepared.

Finances

I manage my finances to benefit me. I manage my food so that my body stays at a healthy weight.

Illusion

The illusion that *smaller is better* is not the right one when it comes to sweets. For example, one chocolate with caramel filling wrapped in sparkly paper is 78 calories! Who can stop at just one? An alternative example: 1 wrapped caramel candy is 25 calories.

Chapter 29

Doomsayers

See it, eat it. Advising people to go through the fridge, freezer and pantry and put food in the bin so that they won't be tempted, is ridiculous. Considering the waste, I have to consider family and visitors that could be coming. There always has to be a selection of food and drink to choose from. I just have to count my calories and prepare my meals carefully.

Chapter 30

Recollections

It had been said you can never be too thin. At 68 kilos when I looked in the mirror, my face was tired and withdrawn. The decision I made was to be happy with 70 kilos and gradually my face and neck filled out. Now I look better and fresher.

Chapter 31

Suggestible Eating.

....

I ask myself is it

- Boredom
- Advertisements
- Television
- Tiredness
- Brain — Fade
- To entertain oneself
- To get a high
- To relieve anxiety
- To calm oneself
- For stress
- De-hydration
- Habitual

I select an exchange

- Drink water
- Lo-cal snack
- Leave the kitchen
- Nap 20 minutes
- Walk outside
- Car — short drive
- Visit charity shops
- Explore a shopping area
- Buy a magazine
- Buy a lottery ticket
- Explore a nursery
- Buy a plant
- Gardening — list tasks
- The park
- The gymnasium
- The swimming pool
- The hairdresser
- The beautician
- Have a manicure
- Have a pedicure
- The library
- Think of others
- Birthdays Easter Christmas

- Housework — list tasks
- Music
- Meditate
- Sit in the sun
- Read a book
- The beach
- Go to bed early

www.ingramcontent.com/pod-product-compliance
Lightning Source LLC
Chambersburg PA
CBHW051248020426
42333CB00025B/3105